Treatment Methods for Kidney Failure
PERITONEAL DIALYSIS

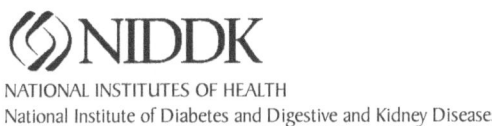

NATIONAL INSTITUTES OF HEALTH
National Institute of Diabetes and Digestive and Kidney Diseases

Contents

Introduction

With peritoneal dialysis (PD), you have some choices in treating advanced and permanent kidney failure. Since the 1980s, when PD first became a practical and widespread treatment for kidney failure, much has been learned about how to make PD more effective and minimize side effects. Since you don't have to schedule dialysis sessions at a center, PD gives you more control. You can give yourself treatments at home, at work, or on trips. But this independence makes it especially important that you work closely with your health care team: your nephrologist, dialysis nurse, dialysis technician, dietitian, and social worker. But the most important members of your health care team are you and your family. By learning about your treatment, you can work with your health care team to give yourself the best possible results, and you can lead a full, active life.

When Your Kidneys Fail

Healthy kidneys clean your blood by removing excess fluid, minerals, and wastes. They also make hormones that keep your bones strong and your blood healthy. When your kidneys fail, harmful wastes build up in your body, your blood pressure may rise, and your body may retain excess fluid and not make enough red blood cells. When this happens, you need treatment to replace the work of your failed kidneys.

How PD Works

In PD, a soft tube called a catheter is used to fill your abdomen with a cleansing liquid called dialysis solution. The walls of your abdominal cavity are lined with a membrane called the peritoneum, which allows waste products and extra fluid to pass from your blood into the dialysis solution. The solution contains a sugar called dextrose that will pull wastes and extra fluid into the abdominal cavity. These wastes and fluid then leave your body when the dialysis solution is drained. The used solution, containing wastes and extra fluid, is then thrown away. The process of draining and filling is called an exchange and takes about 30 to 40 minutes. The period the

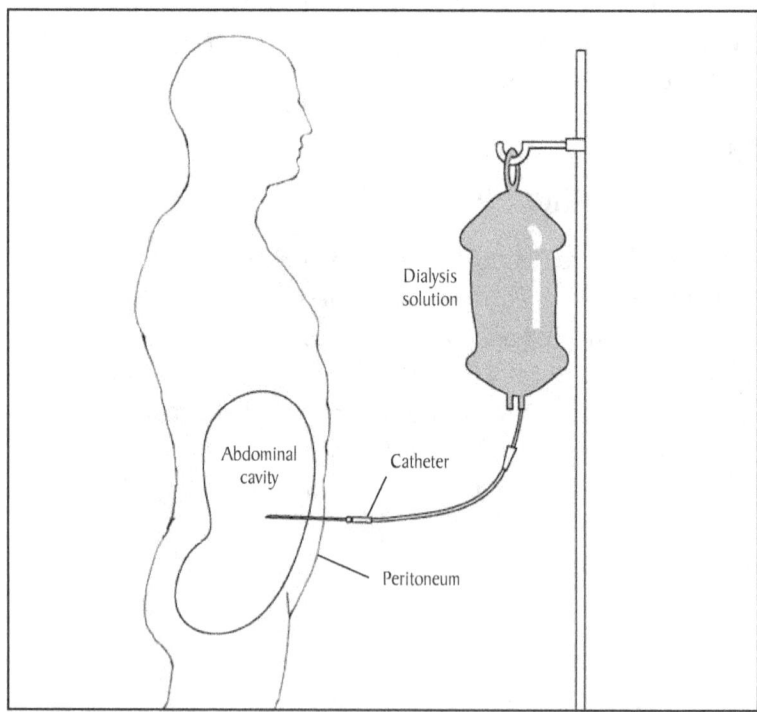

Peritoneal dialysis.

dialysis solution is in your abdomen is called the dwell time. A typical schedule calls for four exchanges a day, each with a dwell time of 4 to 6 hours. Different types of PD have different schedules of daily exchanges.

One form of PD, continuous ambulatory peritoneal dialysis (CAPD), doesn't require a machine. As the word ambulatory suggests, you can walk around with the dialysis solution in your abdomen. Another form of PD, continuous cycler-assisted peritoneal dialysis (CCPD), requires a machine called a cycler to fill and drain your abdomen, usually while you sleep. CCPD is also sometimes called automated peritoneal dialysis (APD).

Getting Ready for PD

Whether you choose an ambulatory or automated form of PD, you'll need to have a soft catheter placed in your abdomen. The catheter is the tube that carries the dialysis solution into and out of your abdomen. If your doctor uses open surgery to insert your catheter, you will be placed under general anesthesia. Another technique requires only local anesthetic. Your doctor will make a small cut, often below and a little to the side of your navel (belly button), and then guide the catheter through the slit into the peritoneal cavity. As soon as the catheter is in place, you can start to receive solution through it, although you probably won't begin a full schedule of exchanges for 2 to 3 weeks. This break-in period lets you build up scar tissue that will hold the catheter in place.

The standard catheter for PD is made of soft tubing for comfort. It has cuffs made of a polyester material, called Dacron, that merge with your scar tissue to keep it in place. The end of the tubing that is inside your abdomen has many holes to allow the free flow of solution in and out.

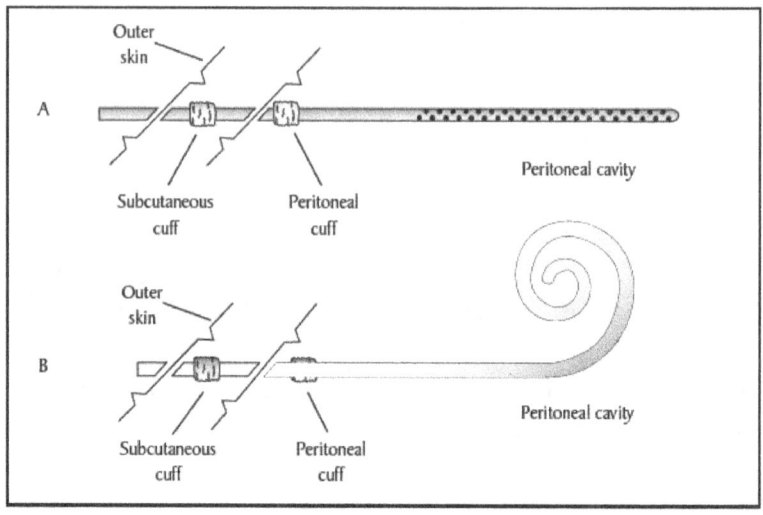

Two double-cuff Tenckhoff peritoneal catheters: standard (A), curled (B).

Types of PD

The type of PD you choose will depend on the schedule of exchanges you would like to follow, as well as other factors. You may start with one type of PD and switch to another, or you may find that a combination of automated and nonautomated exchanges suits you best. Work with your health care team to find the best schedule and techniques to meet your lifestyle and health needs.

Continuous Ambulatory Peritoneal Dialysis (CAPD)

If you choose CAPD, you'll drain a fresh bag of dialysis solution into your abdomen. After 4 to 6 or more hours of dwell time, you'll drain the solution, which now contains wastes, into the bag. You then repeat the cycle with a fresh bag of solution. You don't need a machine for CAPD; all you need is gravity to fill and empty your abdomen. Your doctor will prescribe the number of exchanges you'll need, typically three or four exchanges during the day and one evening exchange with a long overnight dwell time while you sleep.

Continuous Cycler-Assisted Peritoneal Dialysis (CCPD)

CCPD uses an automated cycler to perform three to five exchanges during the night while you sleep. In the morning, you begin one exchange with a dwell time that lasts the entire day.

Customizing Your PD

If you've chosen CAPD, you may have a problem with the long overnight dwell time. It's normal for some of the dextrose in the solution to cross into your body and become glucose. The absorbed dextrose doesn't create a problem during short dwell times. But overnight, some people absorb so much dextrose that it starts to draw fluid from the peritoneal cavity back into the body, reducing the efficiency of the exchange. If you have this problem, you may be able to use a minicycler (a small version of a machine that automatically fills and drains your abdomen) to exchange your solution once or several times overnight while you sleep. These additional, shorter exchanges will minimize solution absorption and give you added clearance of wastes and excess fluid.

If you've chosen CCPD, you may have a solution absorption problem with the daytime exchange, which has a long dwell time. You may find you need an additional exchange in the mid-afternoon to increase the amount of waste removed and to prevent excessive absorption of solution.

Preventing Problems

Infection is the most common problem for people on PD. Your health care team will show you how to keep your catheter bacteria-free to avoid peritonitis, which is an infection of the peritoneum. Improved catheter designs protect against the spread of bacteria, but peritonitis is still a common problem that sometimes makes continuing PD impossible. You should follow your health care team's instructions carefully, but here are some general rules:

- Store supplies in a cool, clean, dry place.

- Inspect each bag of solution for signs of contamination before you use it.

- Find a clean, dry, well-lit space to perform your exchanges.

- Wash your hands every time you need to handle your catheter.

- Clean the exit site with antiseptic every day.

- Wear a surgical mask when performing exchanges.

Keep a close watch for any signs of infection and report them so they can be treated promptly. Here are some signs to watch for:

- Fever

- Nausea or vomiting

- Redness or pain around the catheter

- Unusual color or cloudiness in used dialysis solution

- A catheter cuff that has been pushed out

Equipment and Supplies for PD

Transfer Set

A transfer set is tubing that connects the bag of dialysis solution to the catheter. When your catheter is first placed, the exposed end of the tube will be securely capped to prevent infection. Under the cap is a universal connector.

When you start dialysis training, your dialysis nurse will provide a transfer set. The type of transfer set you receive depends on the company that supplies your dialysis solution. Different companies have different systems for connecting to your catheter.

Connecting the transfer set requires sterile technique. You and your nurse will wear surgical masks. Your nurse will soak the transfer set and the end of your catheter in an antiseptic solution for 5 minutes before making the connection. The nurse will wear rubber gloves while making the connection.

Depending on the company that supplies your solution, your transfer set may require a new cap each time you disconnect from the bag after an exchange. With a different system, the tubing that connects to the transfer set includes a piece that can be clamped at the end of an exchange and then broken off from the tubing so that it stays on the transfer set as a cap until it is removed for the next exchange. Your dialysis nurse will train you in the aseptic (germ-free) technique for connecting at the beginning of an exchange and disconnecting at the end. Follow instructions carefully to avoid infection.

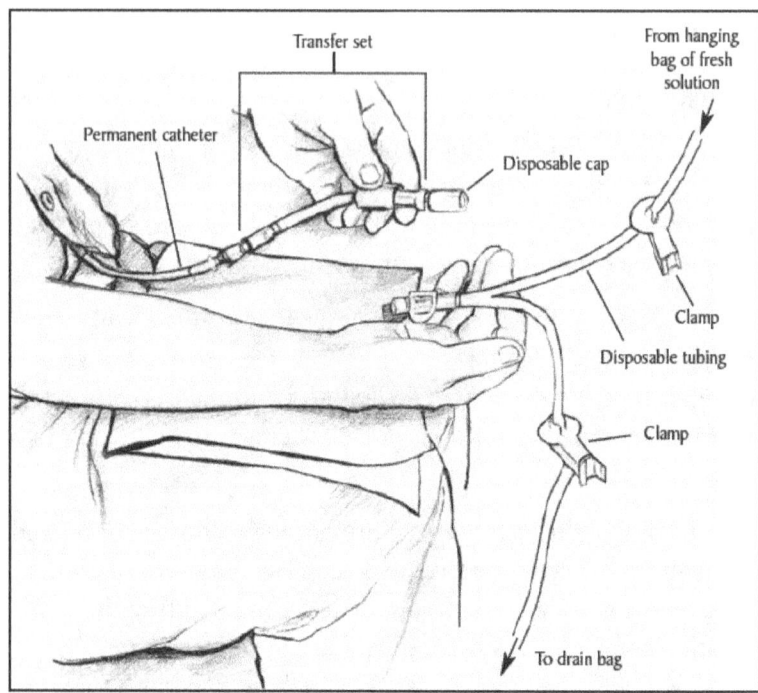

Transfer set. Between exchanges, you can keep your catheter and transfer set hidden inside your clothing. At the beginning of an exchange, you will remove the disposable cap from the transfer set and connect it to a Y-tube. The branches of the Y-tube connect to the drain bag and the bag of fresh dialysis solution. Always wash your hands before handling your catheter and transfer set, and wear a surgical mask whenever you connect or disconnect.

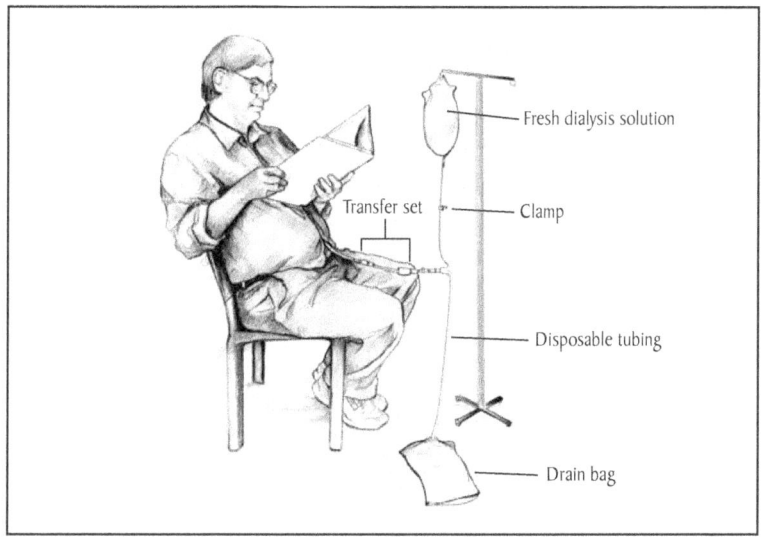

- Fresh dialysis solution
- Transfer set
- Clamp
- Disposable tubing
- Drain bag

During an exchange, you can read, talk, watch television, or sleep.

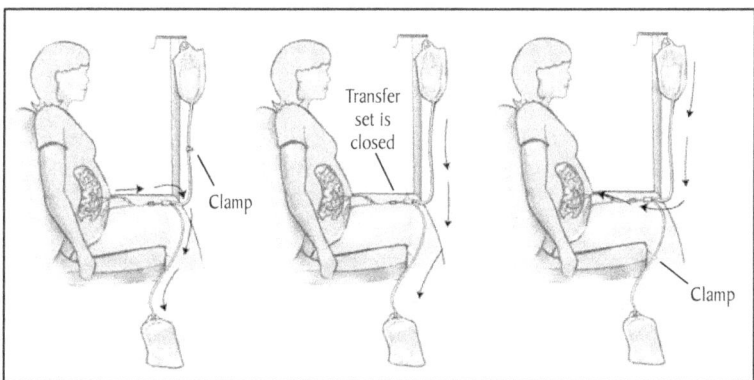

Clamp

Transfer set is closed

Clamp

The first step of an exchange is to drain the used dialysis solution from the peritoneal cavity into the drain bag. Near the end of the drain, you may feel a mild "tugging" sensation that tells you most of your fluid is gone.

After the used solution is removed from your abdomen, you will close or clamp the transfer set and let some of the fresh solution flow directly into the drain bag. This flushing step removes air from the tubes.

The final step of the exchange is to refill the peritoneal cavity with fresh dialysis solution from the hanging bag.

9

Dialysis Solution

Dialysis solution comes in 1.5-, 2-, 2.5-, or 3-liter bags. A liter is slightly more than 1 quart. The dialysis dose can be increased by using a larger bag, but only within the limit of the amount your abdomen can hold. The solution contains a sugar called dextrose, which pulls extra fluid from your blood. Your doctor will prescribe a formula that fits your needs.

You'll need a clean space to store your bags of solution and other supplies. You may also need a special heating device to warm each bag of solution to body temperature before use. Most solution bags come in a protective outer wrapper that allows for microwave heating. Do not microwave a bag of solution after it has been removed from its wrapper because microwaving can change the chemical makeup of the solution.

Cycler

The cycler—which automatically fills and drains your abdomen, usually at night while you sleep—can be programmed to deliver specified volumes of dialysis solution on a specified schedule. Most systems include the following components:

- **Solution storage.** At the beginning of the session, you connect bags of dialysis solution to tubing that feeds the cycler. Most systems include a separate tube for the last bag because this solution may have a higher dextrose content so that it can work for a day-long dwell time.

- **Pump.** The pump sends the solution from the storage bags to the heater bag before it enters the body and then sends it to the disposal container or drain line after it's been used. The pump doesn't fill and drain your abdomen; gravity performs that job more safely.

- **Heater bag.** Before the solution enters your abdomen, a measured dose is warmed to body temperature. Once the solution is the right temperature and the previous exchange has been drained, a clamp is released to allow the warmed solution to flow into your abdomen.

- **Fluid meter.** The cycler's timer releases a clamp to let the used dialysis solution drain from your abdomen into a disposal container or drain line. As the solution flows through the tube, a fluid meter in the cycler measures and records how much solution has been removed. Some systems compare the amount of solution inserted with the amount drained and display the net difference between the two volumes. This lets you know whether the treatment is removing enough fluid from your body.

- **Disposal container or drain line.** After the used solution is weighed, it's pumped to a disposal container that you can throw away in the morning. With some systems, you can dispose of the used fluid directly by stringing a long drain line from the cycler to a toilet or bathtub.

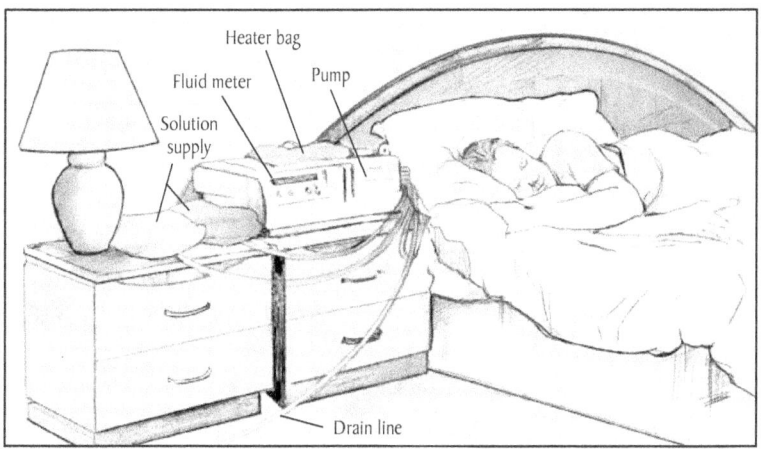

Cycler. A cycler performs four or five exchanges overnight, while you sleep.

- **Alarms.** Sensors will trigger an alarm and shut off the machine if there's a problem with inflow or outflow.

Testing the Effectiveness of Your Dialysis

To see if the exchanges are removing enough waste products, such as urea, your health care team must perform several tests. These tests are especially important during the first weeks of dialysis to determine whether you're receiving an adequate amount, or dose, of dialysis.

The peritoneal equilibration test (often called the PET) measures how much sugar has been absorbed from a bag of infused dialysis solution and how much urea and creatinine have entered into the solution during a 4-hour exchange. The peritoneal transport rate varies from person to person. If you have a high rate of transport, you absorb sugar from the dialysis solution quickly and should avoid exchanges with a very long dwell time because you're likely to absorb too much solution from such exchanges.

In the clearance test, samples of used solution drained over a 24-hour period are collected, and a blood sample is obtained during the day when the used solution is collected. The amount of urea in the used solution is compared with the amount in the blood to see how effective the PD schedule is in removing urea from the blood. For the first months or even years of PD treatment, you may still produce small amounts of urine. If your urine output is more than several hundred milliliters per day, urine is also collected during this period to measure its urea concentration.

From the used solution, urine, and blood measurements, your health care team can compute a urea clearance, called Kt/V, and a creatinine clearance rate (adjusted to body surface area). The residual clearance of the kidneys is also considered. These measurements will show whether the PD prescription is adequate.

If the laboratory results show that the dialysis schedule is not removing enough urea and creatinine, the doctor may change the prescription by

- increasing the number of exchanges per day for patients treated with CAPD or per night for patients treated with CCPD

- increasing the volume of each exchange (amount of solution in the bag) in CAPD

- adding an extra, automated middle-of-the-night exchange to the CAPD schedule

- adding an extra middle-of-the-day exchange to the CCPD schedule

For more information about testing the effectiveness of your dialysis, see the National Institute of Diabetes and Digestive and Kidney Diseases (NIDDK) fact sheet *Peritoneal Dialysis Dose and Adequacy.*

Compliance

One of the big problems with PD is that patients sometimes don't perform all of the exchanges prescribed by their medical team. They either skip exchanges or sometimes skip entire treatment days when using CCPD. Skipping PD treatments has been shown to increase the risk of hospitalization and death.

Remaining Kidney Function

Normally the PD prescription factors in the amount of residual, or remaining, kidney function. Residual kidney function typically falls, although slowly, over months or even years of PD. This means that more often than not, the number of exchanges prescribed, or the volume of exchanges, needs to increase as residual kidney function falls.

The doctor should determine your PD dose on the basis of practice standards established by the National Kidney Foundation Dialysis Outcomes Quality Initiative (NKF-DOQI). Work closely with your health care team to ensure that you get the proper dose, and follow instructions carefully to make sure you get the most out of your dialysis exchanges.

Conditions Related to Kidney Failure and Their Treatments

Your kidneys do much more than remove wastes and extra fluid. They also make hormones and balance chemicals in your system. When your kidneys stop working, you may have problems with anemia and conditions that affect your bones, nerves, and skin. Some of the more common conditions caused by kidney failure are fatigue, bone problems, joint problems, itching, and restless legs.

Anemia and Erythropoietin (EPO)

Anemia is a condition in which the volume of red blood cells is low. Red blood cells carry oxygen to cells throughout the body. Without oxygen, cells can't use the energy from food, so someone with anemia may tire easily and look pale. Anemia can also contribute to heart problems.

Anemia is common in people with kidney disease because the kidneys produce the hormone erythropoietin (EPO), which stimulates the bone marrow to produce red blood cells. Diseased kidneys often don't make enough EPO, and so the bone marrow makes fewer red blood cells. EPO is available commercially and is commonly given to patients on dialysis.

For more information about the causes of and treatments for anemia in kidney failure, see the NIDDK fact sheet *Anemia in Kidney Disease and Dialysis*.

Renal Osteodystrophy

The term "renal" describes things related to the kidneys. Renal osteodystrophy, or bone disease of kidney failure, affects up to 90 percent of dialysis patients. It causes bones to become thin and weak or malformed and affects both children and adults. Symptoms can be seen in growing children with kidney disease even before they start dialysis. Older patients and women who have gone through menopause are at greater risk for this disease.

For more information about the causes of this bone disease and its treatment in dialysis patients, see the NIDDK fact sheet *Renal Osteodystrophy*.

Itching (Pruritus)

Many people treated with peritoneal dialysis complain of itchy skin. Itching is common even in people who don't have kidney disease; with kidney failure, however, itching can be made worse by uremic toxins in the blood that dialysis doesn't adequately remove. The problem can also be related to high levels of parathyroid hormone (PTH). Some people have found dramatic relief after having their parathyroid glands removed. But a cure that works for everyone has not been found. Phosphate binders seem to help some people; others find relief after exposure to ultraviolet light. Still others improve with EPO shots. A few antihistamines (Benadryl, Atarax, Vistaril) have been found to help; also, capsaicin cream applied to the skin may relieve itching by deadening nerve impulses. In any case, taking care of dry skin is important. Applying creams with lanolin or camphor may help.

Sleep Disorders

Patients on dialysis often have insomnia, and some people have a specific problem called sleep apnea syndrome. Episodes of apnea are breaks in breathing during sleep. Over time, these sleep disturbances can lead to "day-night reversal" (insomnia at night, sleepiness during the day), headache, depression, and decreased alertness. The apnea may be related to the effects of advanced kidney failure on the control of breathing. Treatments that work with people who have sleep apnea, whether they have kidney failure or not, include losing weight, changing sleeping position, and wearing a mask that gently pumps air continuously into the nose, called nasal continuous positive airway pressure (CPAP).

Many people on dialysis have trouble sleeping at night because of aching, uncomfortable, jittery, or restless legs. You may feel a strong impulse to kick or thrash your legs. Kicking may occur during sleep and disturb a bed partner throughout the night. Theories about the causes of this syndrome include nerve damage and chemical imbalances.

Moderate exercise during the day may help, but exercising a few hours before bedtime can make it worse. People with restless leg syndrome should reduce or avoid caffeine, alcohol, and tobacco; some people also find relief with massages or warm baths. A class of drugs called benzodiazepines, often used to treat insomnia or anxiety, may help as well. These prescription drugs include Klonopin, Librium, Valium, and Halcion. A newer and sometimes more effective therapy is levodopa (Sinemet), a drug used to treat Parkinson's disease.

Sleep disorders may seem unimportant, but they can impair your quality of life. Don't hesitate to raise these problems with your nurse, doctor, or social worker.

Amyloidosis

Dialysis-related amyloidosis (DRA) is common in people who have been on dialysis for more than 5 years. DRA develops when proteins in the blood deposit on joints and tendons, causing pain, stiffness, and fluid in the joints, as is the case with arthritis. Working kidneys filter out these proteins, but dialysis is not as effective. For more information, see the NIDDK fact sheet *Amyloidosis and Kidney Disease.*

Adjusting to Changes

You can do your exchanges in any clean space, and you can take part in many activities with solution in your abdomen. Even though PD gives you more flexibility and freedom than hemodialysis, which requires being connected to a machine for 3 to 5 hours three times a week, you must still stick to a strict schedule of exchanges and keep track of supplies. You may have to cut back on some responsibilities at work or in your home life. Accepting this new reality can be very hard on you and your family. A counselor or social worker can help you cope.

Many patients feel depressed when starting dialysis, or after several months of treatment. Some people can't get used to the fact that the solution makes their body look larger. If you feel depressed, you should talk with your social worker, nurse, or doctor because depression is a common problem that can often be treated effectively.

How Diet Can Help

Eating the right foods can help improve your dialysis and your health. You may have chosen PD over hemodialysis because the diet is less restrictive. With PD, you're removing wastes from your body slowly but constantly, while in hemodialysis, wastes may build up for 2 or 3 days between treatments. You still need to be very careful about the foods you eat, however, because PD is much less efficient than working kidneys. Your clinic has a dietitian to help you plan meals. Follow the dietitian's advice closely to get the most from your dialysis treatments. You can also ask your dietitian for recipes and titles of cookbooks for patients with kidney disease. Following the restrictions of a diet for kidney failure might be hard at first, but with a little creativity, you can make tasty and satisfying meals.

The National Kidney Foundation has a brochure on *Nutrition and Peritoneal Dialysis,* which gives general guidelines on calorie and nutrient intake. See the "Additional Reading" section for contact information.

Financial Issues

Treatment for kidney failure is expensive, but Federal health insurance programs pay much of the cost, usually up to 80 percent. Often, private insurance or State programs pay the rest. Your social worker can help you locate resources for financial assistance. For more information, see the NIDDK fact sheet *Financial Help for Treatment of Kidney Failure.*

Hope Through Research

The NIDDK, through its Division of Kidney, Urologic, and Hematologic Diseases, supports several programs and studies devoted to improving treatment for patients with progressive kidney disease and permanent kidney failure, including patients on PD.

• **The End-Stage Renal Disease Program** promotes research to reduce medical problems from bone, blood, nervous system, metabolic, gastrointestinal, cardiovascular, and endocrine abnormalities in kidney failure and to improve the effectiveness of dialysis and transplantation. The research focuses on reusing hemodialysis membranes and using alternative dialyzer sterilization methods; devising more efficient, biocompatible membranes; refining high-flux hemodialysis; and developing criteria for dialysis adequacy. The program also seeks to increase kidney graft and patient survival and to maximize quality of life.

• The U.S. Renal Data System (USRDS) collects, analyzes, and distributes information about the use of dialysis and transplantation to treat kidney failure in the United States. The USRDS is funded directly by the NIDDK in conjunction with the Health Care Financing Administration. The USRDS publishes an *Annual Data Report,* which characterizes the total population of people being treated for kidney failure; reports on incidence, prevalence, mortality rates, and trends over time; and develops data on the effects of various treatment modalities. The report also helps identify problems and opportunities for more focused special studies of renal research issues.

Resources

Organizations That Can Help

American Association of Kidney Patients
3505 East Frontage Road
Suite 315
Tampa, FL 33607
Phone: 1–800–749–2257
Email: info@aakp.org
Internet: www.aakp.org

American Kidney Fund
6110 Executive Boulevard
Suite 1010
Rockville, MD 20852
Phone: 1–800–638–8299
Email: helpline@kidneyfund.org
Internet: www.kidneyfund.org

Life Options Rehabilitation Program
c/o Medical Education Institute Inc.
414 D'Onofrio Drive
Suite 200
Madison, WI 53711–1074
Phone: 1–800–468–7777
Email: lifeoptions@MEIresearch.org
Internet: www.lifeoptions.org
        www.kidneyschool.org

National Kidney Foundation, Inc.
30 East 33rd Street
New York, NY 10016
Phone: 1–800–622–9010 or 212–889–2210
Email: info@kidney.org
Internet: www.kidney.org

Additional Reading

If you would like to learn more about kidney failure and its treatment, you may be interested in reading the following:

AAKP Patient Plan
This is a series of booklets and newsletters that cover the different phases of learning about kidney failure, choosing a treatment, and adjusting to changes.
American Association of Kidney Patients
3505 East Frontage Road
Suite 315
Tampa, FL 33607
Phone: 1–800–749–2257
Email: info@aakp.org
Internet: www.aakp.org

Getting the Most From Your Treatment series
This is a series of brochures based on the National Kidney Foundation's Dialysis Outcomes Quality Initiative (NKF–DOQI). Titles include *What You Need To Know About Peritoneal Dialysis, What You Need To Know Before Starting Dialysis,* and *What You Need To Know About Anemia.*
Additional patient education brochures include information on diet, work, and exercise.
National Kidney Foundation, Inc.
30 East 33rd Street
New York, NY 10016
Phone: 1–800–622–9010 or 212–889–2210
Email: info@kidney.org
Internet: www.kidney.org

Medicare Coverage of Kidney Dialysis and
Kidney Transplant Services
Publication Number CMS–10128
U.S. Department of Health and Human Services
7500 Security Boulevard
Baltimore, MD 21244–1850
Phone: 1–800–MEDICARE (1–800–633–4227)
TDD: 1–877–486–2048
Internet:
   www.medicare.gov/publications/pubs/pdf/esrdcoverage.pdf

Nutrition and Peritoneal Dialysis
National Kidney Foundation, Inc.
30 East 33rd Street
New York, NY 10016
Phone: 1–800–622–9010 or 212–889–2210
Email: info@kidney.org
Internet: www.kidney.org

Newsletters and Magazines

Family Focus Newsletter (published quarterly)
National Kidney Foundation, Inc.
30 East 33rd Street
New York, NY 10016
Phone: 1–800–622–9010 or 212–889–2210
Email: info@kidney.org
Internet: www.kidney.org

For Patients Only (published six times a year)
ATTN: Subscription Department
18 East 41st Street
20th Floor
New York, NY 10017–6222

Renalife (published quarterly)
American Association of Kidney Patients
3505 East Frontage Road
Suite 315
Tampa, FL 33607
Phone: 1–800–749–2257
Email: info@aakp.org
Internet: www.aakp.org

Acknowledgments

The National Institute of Diabetes and Digestive and Kidney Diseases thanks these dedicated health professionals for their careful review of this publication.

John M. Burkart, M.D.
Wake Forest University Baptist Medical Center

Karl D. Nolph, M.D.
University of Missouri School of Medicine

The individuals listed here facilitated field-testing for this publication. The NIDDK thanks them for their contribution.

Kim Bayer, M.A., R.D., L.D.
BMA Dialysis
Bethesda, MD

Cora Benedicto, R.N.
Clinic Director
Gambro Health Care
N Street Clinic
Washington, DC

About the Kidney Failure Series

You and your doctor will work together to choose a treatment that's best for you. The booklets and fact sheets of the NIDDK Kidney Failure Series can help inform you about the specific issues you will face.

Booklets

- *Kidney Failure: Choosing a Treatment That's Right for You*
- *Treatment Methods for Kidney Failure: Hemodialysis*
- *Treatment Methods for Kidney Failure: Peritoneal Dialysis*
- *Treatment Methods for Kidney Failure: Transplantation*
- *Eat Right to Feel Right on Hemodialysis*
- *Kidney Failure Glossary*

Fact Sheets

- *Kidney Failure: What to Expect*
- *Vascular Access for Hemodialysis*
- *Hemodialysis Dose and Adequacy*
- *Peritoneal Dialysis Dose and Adequacy*
- *Amyloidosis and Kidney Disease*
- *Anemia in Kidney Disease and Dialysis*
- *Renal Osteodystrophy*
- *Financial Help for Treatment of Kidney Failure*

Learning as much as you can about your treatment will help make you an important member of your health care team.

The NIDDK will develop additional materials for this series as needed. Please address any comments about this series and requests for copies to the National Kidney and Urologic Diseases Information Clearinghouse. Descriptions of the publications in this series are available at *www.kidney.niddk. nih.gov/kudiseases/pubs/kidneyfailure/index.htm.*

National Kidney and Urologic Diseases Information Clearinghouse

3 Information Way
Bethesda, MD 20892–3580
Phone: 1–800–891–5390
Fax: 703–738–4929
Email: nkudic@info.niddk.nih.gov
Internet: www.kidney.niddk.nih.gov

The National Kidney and Urologic Diseases Information Clearinghouse (NKUDIC) is a service of the National Institute of Diabetes and Digestive and Kidney Diseases (NIDDK). The NIDDK is part of the National Institutes of Health under the U.S. Department of Health and Human Services. Established in 1987, the Clearinghouse provides information about diseases of the kidneys and urologic system to people with kidney and urologic disorders and to their families, health care professionals, and the public. The NKUDIC answers inquiries, develops and distributes publications, and works closely with professional and patient organizations and Government agencies to coordinate resources about kidney and urologic diseases.

Publications produced by the Clearinghouse are carefully reviewed by both NIDDK scientists and outside experts.